Cancer Glue for Caregivers

Give & Accept Help, & Protect Yourself

Reverend Mike Wanner

Copyright
Rev. Mike Wanner
July 9, 2019

Selected Images Used by License

Table of Contents

Introduction

When I was a child, my father got sick with cancer, and he had a hard time, and eventually, God called him, and I missed him. That was many years ago, and I wished that I could have done more for him.

I did not understand, but I wanted to, and it was impossible to know what to do to help others. I tried to comprehend but could not find answers.

Wanting to understand has influenced my life. The one thing that I remembered so firmly was the importance of kindness.

While kindness to others is relatively easy, being kind to oneself can be a big challenge. Many have accumulated unkind views of themselves and their situations that can repeat self-hurt until changed.

Choosing new scripts can be transformational, please consider what you have allowed and when you want to change.

I dedicate this book to everybody living in these chaotic times who wish to optimize their control over their conscious awareness of any programming that may best be updated.

1 - Why I Am Writing This Book

After many decades in the back of an ambulance giving patient care and a lot more time now at the bedside doing Pastoral Care, I have seen and heard a lot of situations. Caregivers are usually well respected by the medical community.

The story least told is about the challenges of Care Giving. It is a lot of work, and it is not always appreciated or rewarded.

Different family cultures can have patterns which can burn out a caregiver in the short term and have long term consequences for the family and their finances,

"Many hands make light work" is an old expression that is still true today. Balance can be essential to sustain a long term pattern of care that is participated in by the whole family.

The tendency in families may be to let some individuals have the burden of the work. Unfortunately, many times, the individual chosen is a female who may not be physically able to do some of the tasks that need doing.

Taking care of an ill or injured family member is a family challenge, and it is imperative to involve as many people as possible in the remedy needed.

The whole family can be severely stressed impacted if there is not a reasonably well-developed answer to caregiving issues.

2 - Sharing In The Work Can Be Satisfying

When a person does their fair share of the work on a project, they are entitled to feel good about all they have contributed. So, it makes sense that all family members be asked to do a reasonable share. What is it that each can do best and would not mind doing the least?

A lot of people nowadays have mobile devices, and they can work freely in many locations. This mobility can be an advantage for families who have patients in need of care.

Family members who can work anywhere can plan to be with their family member patient a day or two or three each week so that primary caregivers can get a break and go out and get things they need to do done.

Scheduling these mental health breaks in advance creates a real stress reduction for the primary caregiver.

Meal preparation can be another area where support can be optimized. People in the family who are less able to be present for the day-to-day care can still do meal preparation to shorten the list of duties for the primary caregiver.

Every little bit of help can make a difference in the size of the primary caregiver's efforts agenda and can also act as psychological support to both the caregiver and the Cancer patient.

3 - Cancer Care is A Deep Subject

As I go along with my general hospital ministry, the information flowing to me is quite staggering in size and complexity. A lot is going on in the minds of patients and their caregivers.

The most terrible things that I hear is about the energy of the patients being minimal, the patience being lacking, and the fear being constant and excessive. I keep reflecting on the fact that fear and worry may be at least as catastrophic as the disease.

The fear creates the appearance of an impenetrable force that cannot be tamed. The image looms significant and stimulates disturbing images that can rattle otherwise quiet minds.

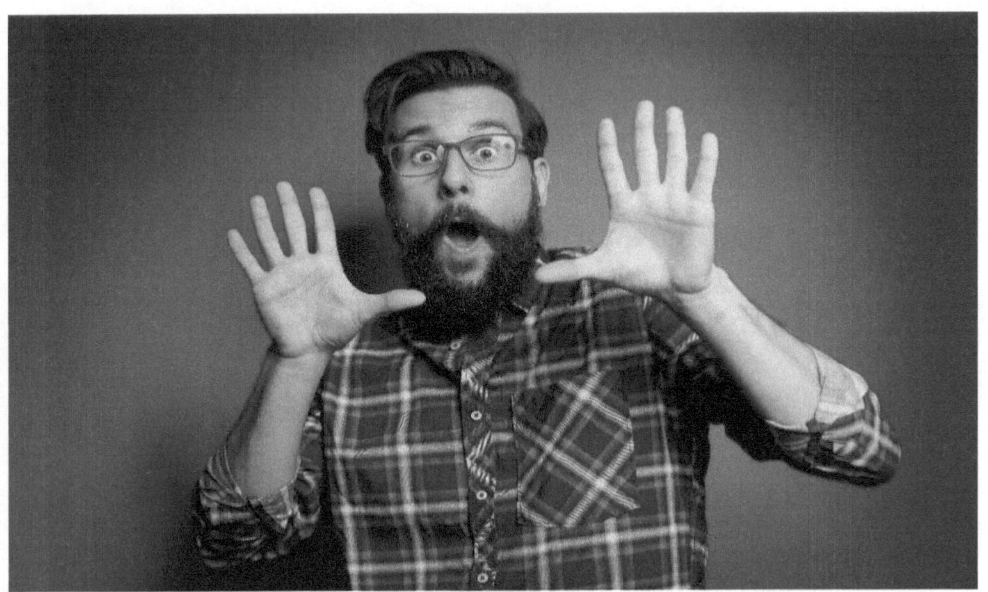

A Cancer Diagnosis is A Real Loud Alarm Bell For the Patient

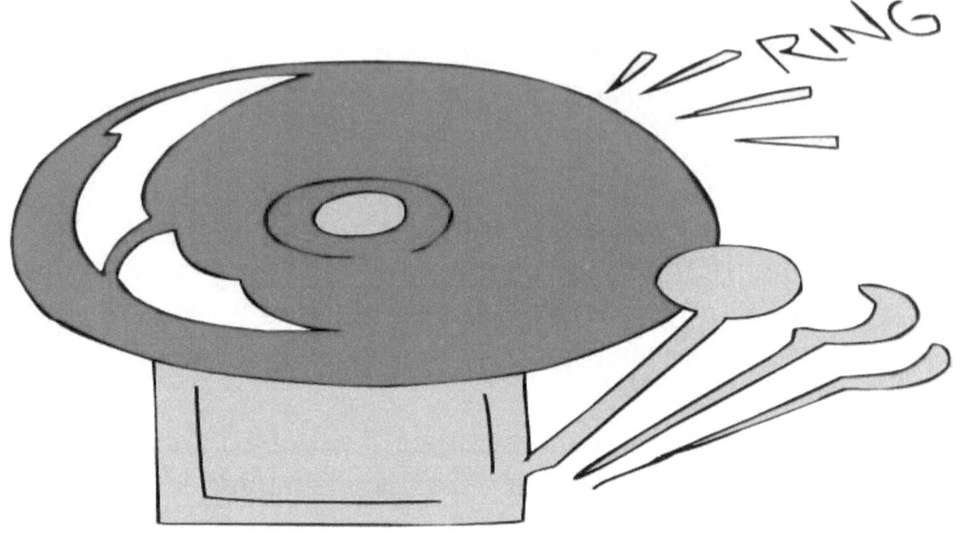

Pain Calls For Attention.
Many Basic Changes Maybe Needed.

Please Consider Optimizing:

Physical Change/Support

Emotional Change/Support

Mental Change/Support

Spiritual Change/Support

4 - Caregivers Role In Support

The primary role of the caregiver is like the Maestro conducting an orchestra. It all about the big picture and keeping the process harmonious for the patient, the family members, the doctors, the nurses, the technicians, the support staff, transport personnel and all those who are interacting with the patient.

The primary caregivers are human beings, and the oversight that can affect the patient is a difficult task at least. Trying to do all the negotiating of time and talent and schedules is a Herculean task, and the ability to do it all requires that the caregivers accept and orchestrate all the help they can get.

The finesse needed by caregivers will require dedication because getting people motivated is not an exact science, and creativity will be critical to success.

In the next chapters, I will bring up things for caregiver consideration, some of which may not make sense. When you can't logically accept a suggestion, I invite you to ask within the question – "If not this, then what will get the same result?"

The last chapter will be about protecting yourself because all who help others can become vulnerable to the one who they are trying so hard to support. Stay aware please and ask for all the help you need, because asking for and receiving support is essential to your success.

5 - Welcome Friends to BYO Meal

Friends Can Bring The Meal For the One Needing Care and Eat It With Them.

How many times have you heard people say, "Let me know if there is anything that I can do for him/her or you." And what happens? Not much, usually.

Let's change that. Say well; you could schedule with me (the caregiver) a block of time where you could bring a meal (lunch or dinner) and heat it and sit down with him/her and visit and eat together.

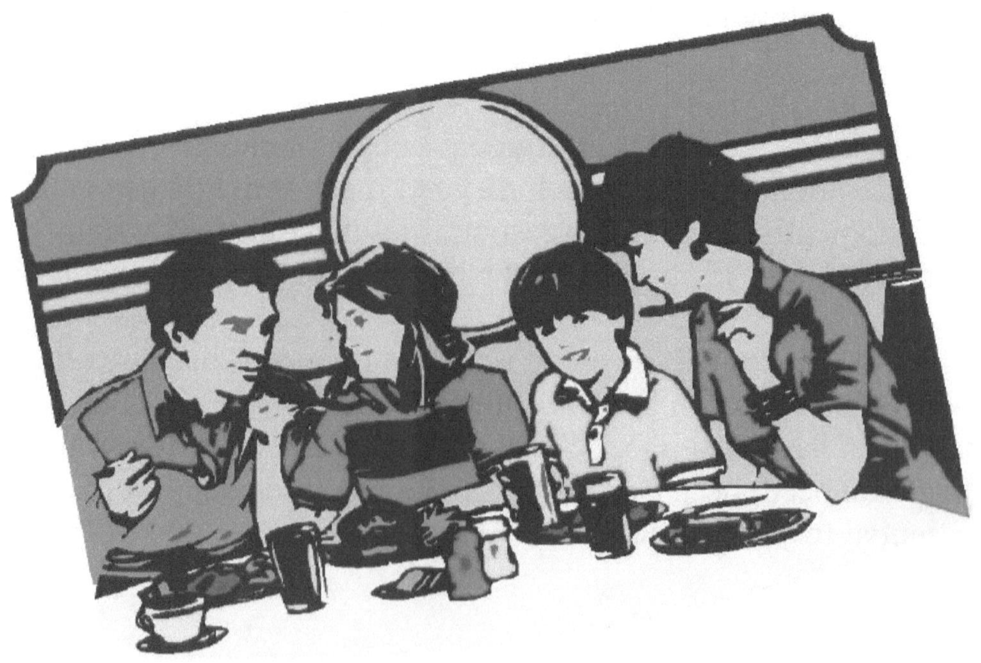

A visit that is two to three hours long could help a caregiver a lot by being a mini-vacation and a change of scenery. The same visit could help the patient a lot by having a bit of normality where the audience was fresh and wanting to share their life even during the difficult time they are facing.

The informality and break in the pattern of regular life can add excellent value to the life of the patient as it destresses the living arrangement for both the patient and the caregiver.

Some patients may share essential information with their friends that could help caregivers and the care team know how to simplify the needed care.

Visitors could be considerate and save a portion of the meal for the caregiver when they return. Visitors can walk away from visiting their friend and know that they made both a statement of their support and a real difference in showing what support does for optimizing the situation.

6 - Caregivers "Little Help Please" List

Often you will hear men talking about their "Honey Do" List, and they are not referring to a melon. They are referring to the list of projects that their spouse wants them to do.

Please consider having a Little Help Needed List for caregivers they can add to when answering questions about the wellness of the one in care. If the caregiver sends the family a status update, this list could be attached to it.

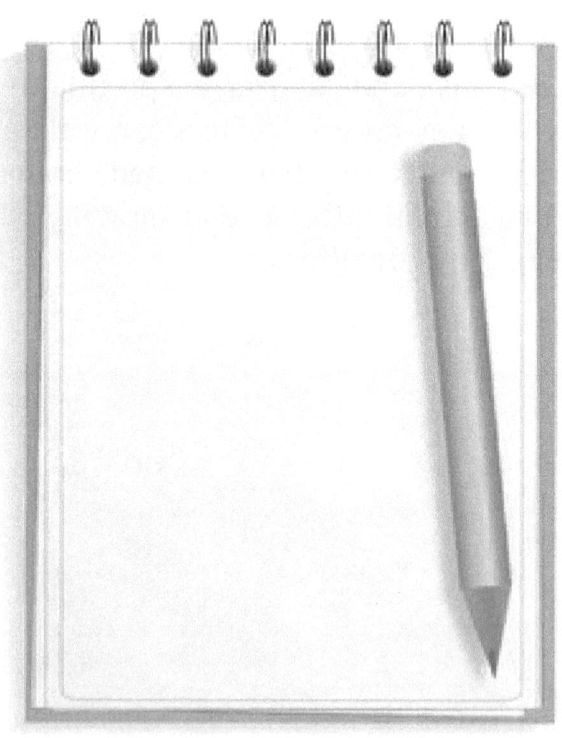

7 - Friends Might Help Patients Get to the Doctor

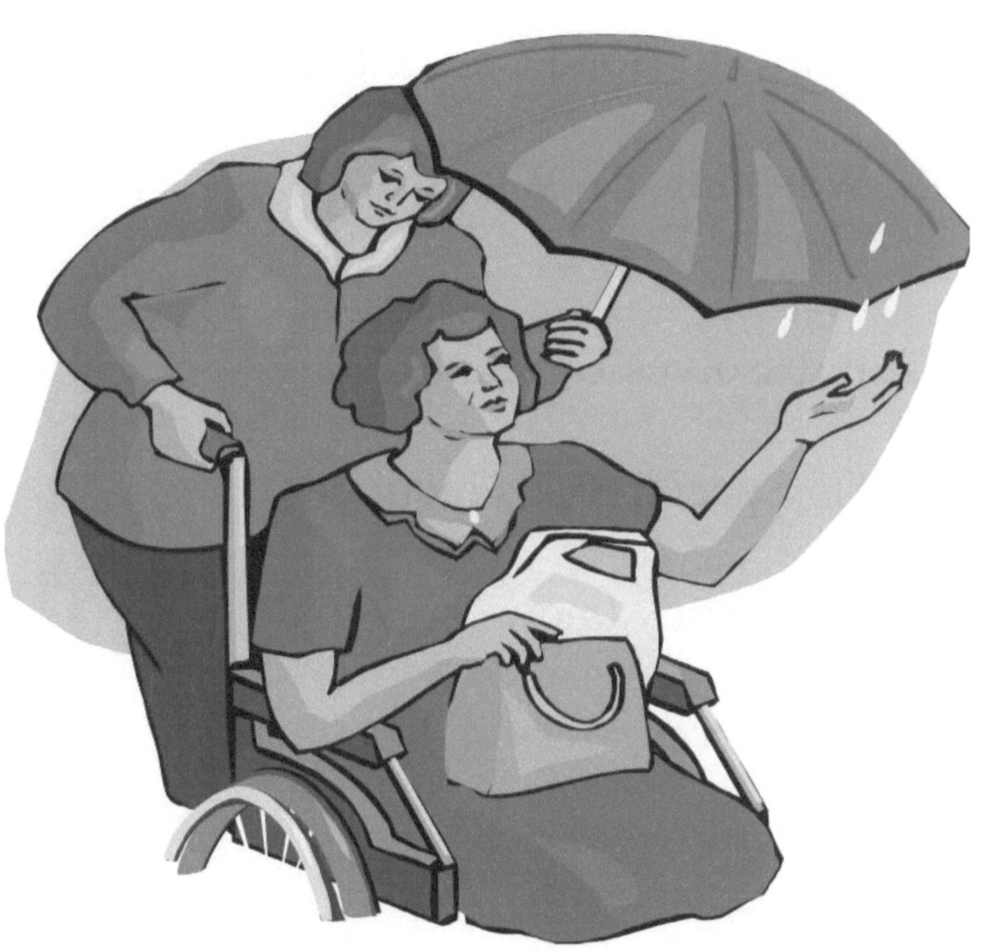

8 - Friends Can Come and Watch TV With Their Friend

Time to Bond Can be a Big Help!

1. Watching TV With Friends Is A Very Normal Event

2. It dissolves Loneliness

3. No Special Skills required

4. Everybody knows how to do it

5. It resolves stress and isolation

9 - Invite The Patient's Prayer Family

Caregivers may not be a church person, so may not think to call the church to which the ill patient goes. Please consider it.

Inviting the church (If the ill one would like it) could be another way to involve friends that support the patient on the mend.

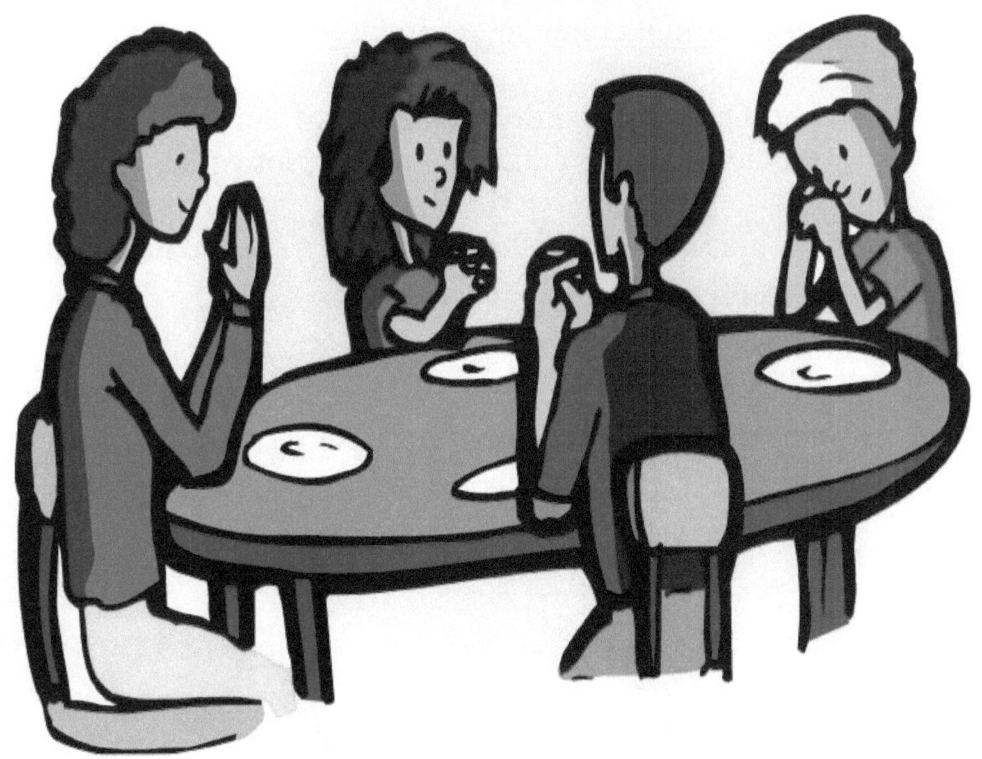

The Ill person gets more support, the caregivers get a break, and the church members get a prayer purpose.

10 - More Prayer Support

On-Line Prayer Request Links

Circle Of Miracles
https://circleofmiracles.org/services/prayer-request/

The Center Of Being, Inc. (Integrated Energy Therapy)
https://www.learniet.com/angel-ariel/need-angelic-support/

The Theosophical Society Order of Service
manages a free of charge Healing Network:

1. For People http://www.theoservice.org/special/names-by-email.shtml

2. For Animals https://www.theoservice.org/spec.../animal-healing-names.shtml

Prayer Resources

http://Create-A-Prayer.com

https://www.prayers.co.uk/

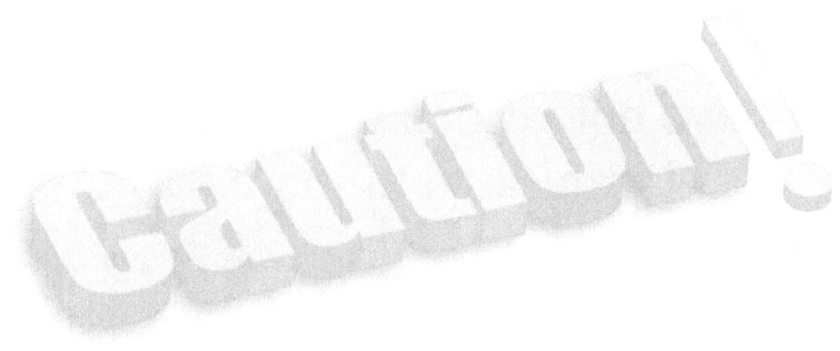

Balance Is Needed
The Needs of The Patient And Your needs
Must be Balanced To Be Healthy

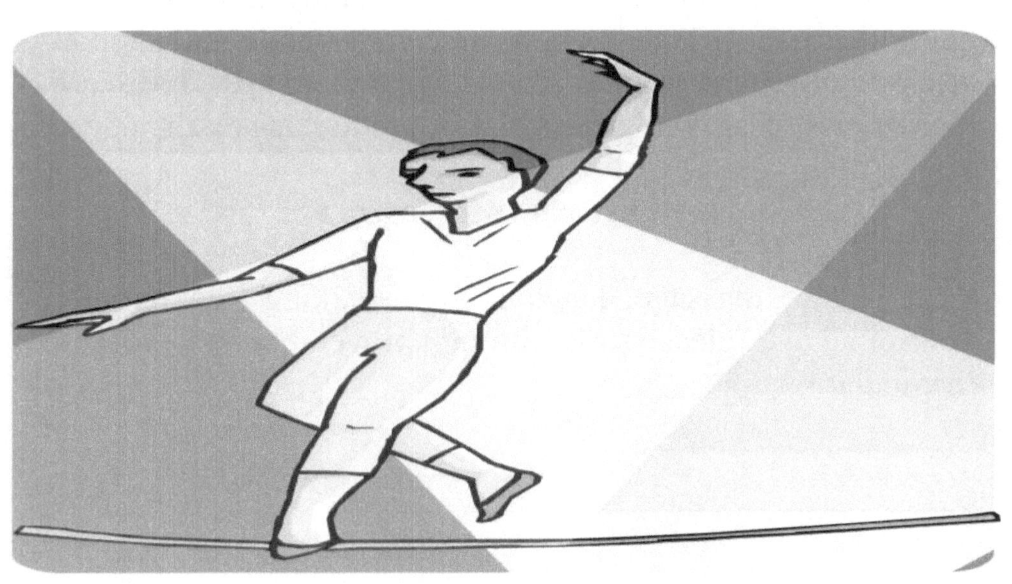

12 - Tips for Caregiver's Coping with Stress and Guilt
(Anonymous Author)

I have not written this, but I have Permission to share it.

Get Support

If you have no friends to talk to who understand what you're going through, then try a 12-step group such as Co-dependents Anonymous.

The meetings are free. A small donation is requested to pay for expenses. The sessions are a safe place to share your feelings without being attacked or judged. It is healing and validating to have other people listen to you share your opinions with total acceptance. CoDA.org has a list of local meetings. There are many types of 12 step groups. There are listings on the internet.

Physical Intervention

Acupuncture, massage, dancing, yoga, walking – get out of your mind and release stress through movement and manipulation.

Mental Therapy

Talk to a counselor/therapist – It helps to have someone who can listen and support you in taking care of yourself.

Energy Work

Energy Work is a great way to get into a deeply relaxed state and to release pent-up stress, fear, and guilt. Energy healing helps strengthen you and brings a sense of inner peace. Reiki and Integrated Energy Therapy are healing modalities that help you release negative emotions and beliefs. This release creates space for a higher vibration of love and light to come in. The release empowers you to create a life that allows you to have the happiness you desire.

Spiritual Counseling

A spiritual counselor helps you understand that you are loved and supported and that you deserve happiness. Spiritual counseling enables you to gain insight into your situation so that you can see more possibilities for positively dealing with your job. Spirituality opens you to your inner strength through divine guidance.

13 - Little Stories That Could Be A Concern
(Anonymous Author)

I have not written these stories, but I have permission to share them.

Story # 1

Being abused by the person you are caring for is more common than you might suspect. The caregiver feels too guilty to complain to anyone about the treatment they receive. I went to someone I thought was a good friend to confide in him and receive healing. He is a Shaman. He scolded me and said, "he has cancer; you have to accept that!" I never went to him again for healing.

Story # 2

I know of another woman who was being abused by her husband, who has cancer. Many years ago, I was a support caregiver for my boyfriend's mom, who was dying of cancer. I heard her verbally abuse her husband every day. I lived with them for two weeks. I was there to comfort him as much as I was there for her. It was heartbreaking. I'm probably the only person who witnessed that.

14 - Big Story
(Anonymous Author)

The Finding Peace While Providing Support For a Loved One With Cancer

I have not written this story, but I have permission to share it.

If you provide emotional and financial support to a significant other who has cancer, there is likely almost no support for you. All the resources and energy go for the person with cancer. Everyone around you asks about your significant other with little thought about how you are managing all the stress and fear that comes with living with someone with cancer.

If your loved one abuses you, there is even less support. Your friends and family don't want to believe that someone with cancer is mean and abusive. You feel guilty for also telling anyone about it.

I offer several tools and techniques (Chapter 12) to help you cope and stay positive through the difficult situation of living with someone who has cancer. I can teach you methods to help you relax and nurture yourself.

My Story

I divorced a man with stage IV cancer. While we were together, I was his most reliable source of support and love. It was hard knowing he could die at any time. We could not plan for the future. In public, he was friendly, charming, and he told our friends how much he loved me.

In private, I felt his fear. I endured his angry attacks and his attempts to control me. I felt guilty every time we fought. I struggled with the guilt of wanting to leave my husband.

It has been over four years since we parted. I had to be strong for so many years. A few years ago, I went through the cleansing process of crying to let go of the deep emotional pain of being in an abusive marriage.

My ex-husband and I managed to stay friends. We have a lot of mutual friends, and my family still loves him. I have healed from the past and live a peaceful life.

Many of you are in the same situation I was. All the money goes toward treatment, and you find yourself giving most of your energy attempting to be tolerant and understanding of the behaviors that go along with the illness.

Your loved one is afraid, angry, and desperate to get control of his or her life. They may be able to present a strong front in public, but you see what is going on privately. It is heartbreaking and hard to endure. You want to help in any way you can.

In the meantime, you have stopped doing most of the things you enjoy, and your relationships with friends and family are stressed. They can't possibly understand what you are going through unless they have lived it. It's not their fault, but that doesn't ease your isolation. You are not sleeping or eating well.

You are desperate to rid yourself of the heartache and pain you are feeling. Exhaustion has set in from focusing entirely on your significant other, and you have lost touch with your own needs and desires.

You deserve to be happy. It is not wrong to put your happiness first. Only you have the power to set boundaries with your loved one so that you can maintain balance in your life.

You are compassionate and loving regardless of how this all turns out. You're still a righteous person. You can begin a journey to rediscover who you once were. You can regain the confidence to rebuild your life and thrive. At this point in the original, the author said she would share some ways to help you cope and to find yourself again and all that is published as Chapter 12 in this book.

15 - Wrap Up

The Caregiver is the most crucial day-to-day support for the patient as the timeliness and integration of the care is heavily dependent on reporting and effectiveness and timing and communication.

Caregivers deserve respect and appreciation. Family members who participate less than the caregiver would be wise to be cautious about critiquing anything that they do not want to do themselves or pay somebody else to do.

Physical Change/Support, Emotional Change/Support, Mental Change/Support and Spiritual Change/Support mentioned above is not detailed here, but page 26 lists books with many ideas to help. Those same books rotate free on the Kindle "Healing Presents" Book Giveaway referenced on page 2.

May all who read this book be blessed, AND SO IT IS!

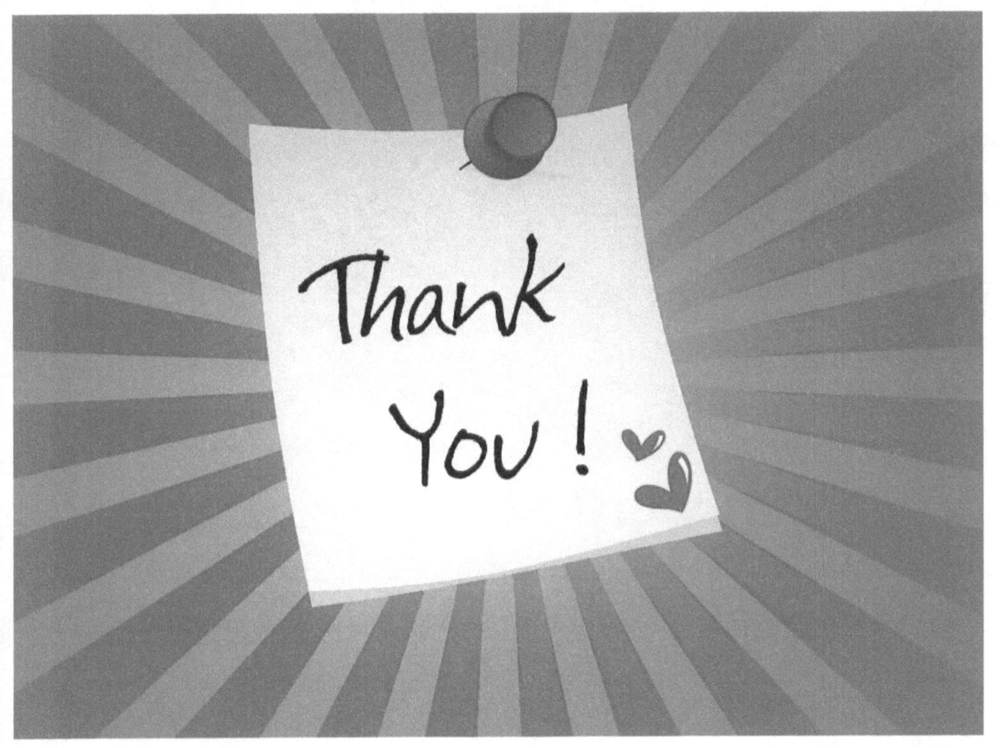

For
Considering
These
Ideas

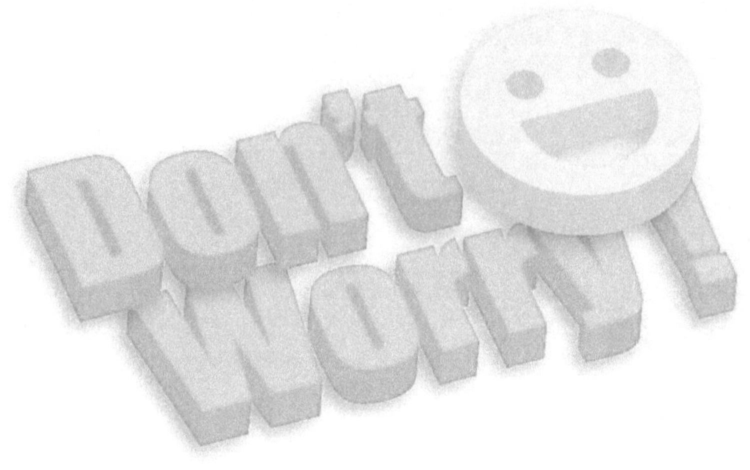

Ever

It Does Not Help Prayer Still Does!

18 - Other Cancer Books by Rev. Mike

Cancer Emotional And Spiritual Compendium: Caring To Support Cancer Care
http://amzn.com/B07N9XYF9R

Cancer Emotional And Spiritual Compendium Volume Two: Caring From An Earlier Time Plus Recent & New Books
http://amzn.com/B07RZD37TM

Does Reiki Love Heal Cancer?: Transcribed True Stories Of Spiritual Healing
http://amzn.com/B00MS6M77I

Reiki Help For Cancer Care in Pottstown, PA: Cecilia Appreciates PMMC Cancer Center
http://amzn.com/B071XBTSFX

Reiki For Cancer
http://amzn.com/B07873YKLJ

Love Energy Circuit Healing For Cancer Patients: Energize & Bond
http://amzn.com/B07QPWGXM1

Cancer Patient's Self-Talk And Reflections: Think High Vibration!
http://amzn.com/B07R7YLNWR

Cancer Glue For Adults: Love From Kids
http://amzn.com/B07JMK6FWG

Cancer Glue For Adults: Love From Reiki
http://amzn.com/B07JQPBWW6

Cancer Glue For You: Family Energy
http://amzn.com/B07KM92DMD

Cancer Glue For Miracles: Believing & Preparing & Expecting
http://amzn.com/B07MHK4XZ2

Cancer Glue For Possibilities: Dowsing Power
http://amzn.com/B07M74L8DV

19 - Books Category Resources
at www.Amazon.com

Distant Healing (or Mail List) e-mail mikewann@voicenet.com

Veterans Healing Six Pack plus 2
http://angelraphaelspeaks.com/healing-books/veterans/

PTSD Power Pack
http://angelraphaelspeaks.com/healing-books/ptsd/

Angel Raphael Speaks Series & Other Angel Books
http://angelraphaelspeaks.com/

Reiki
http://angelraphaelspeaks.com/healing-books/reiki/

Children
http://angelraphaelspeaks.com/healing-books/children/

Emergency Medical Kindness
http://angelraphaelspeaks.com/healing-books/emergency-medical-kindness/

Cancer
http://angelraphaelspeaks.com/healing-books/cancer/

Addictions
http://angelraphaelspeaks.com/healing-books/addictions/

Miscellaneous Healing
http://angelraphaelspeaks.com/healing-books/misc-healing/

Prison Books - 60+ Prison Books
http://angelraphaelspeaks.com/prison-books/

20 - Angels Please Prayers For Addiction

Addict's

Angels of Healing Selected
Help Me to Stay Directed
Come To Me From The Sky
I Am Ready to Succeed Not Try
If I Don't Invite You In
I Might Not Win
I Have Been Lost For Too Long
Help Me To Stay Strong

Alcoholic's

Angels of Healing On High
Help Me to Stay Dry
Come To Me From The Sky
I Am Ready to Succeed Not Try
If I Don't Invite You In
I Might Not Win
I Have Been Lost For Too Long
Help Me To Stay Strong

Prayers Above From

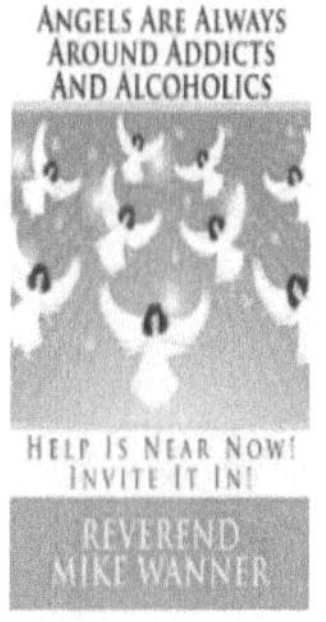

http://AngelRaphaelSpeaks.com/AAAAAAA/
The Link Above Has the Core Messages from the book on drop-down pages.

21 - Private Channeling

Angel Raphael Speaks, a series of free messages channeled through Reverend Mike Wanner for the Highest good and Highest Healing of all concerned.

Many questions arise about Reverend Mike doing private channeling, and he does help with that so E-mail him.

Reverend Mike is available worldwide as a psychic channel, emotional release facilitator, spiritual energy practitioner & teacher, and public speaker.

He looks forward to meeting you soon! Email - mikewann@voicenet.com 215-342-1270

PRIVATE SPIRITUAL READINGS/channelings or Spiritual Healing Sessions can be by telephone or in-person.

Rev. Mike is available for individual, intuitive one-on-one sessions with you, his Guide Family, and your Guides. He helps by offering clarity on emotional situations about your life, your purpose, your spirituality, and your release of stuffed emotions and cellular memory.

Connect to the love of your Guides today!

For more information, please visit
http://angelraphaelspeaks.com/channel/

22 - Reverend Mike Wanner

Rev. Mike Wanner started his spiritual and ministerial studies with Reiki in 1993 and had studied seven styles of Reiki in the U.S., Japan, Canada, Denmark, and Australia. He is certified to teach.

He became certified to teach Integrated Energy Therapy in 1999 and co-taught the first IET class of the new Millennium. Mike began dowsing in 2001.

Ordained as an Interfaith Minister of the Circle of Miracles Ministry and a Metaphysical Minister of the International Metaphysical Ministry, Rev. Mike practices and teaches spiritual energy therapies in the Philadelphia Area.

Rev. Mike holds ministerial degrees from the University of Metaphysics and the University of Sedona. He is a Pastoral Care Associate at Jefferson - Frankford Hospital. He taught at the National Academy of Massage Therapy and Health Sciences.

Rev. Mike was a faculty member of the Medical Mission Sister's Center for Human Integration's School of Integrated Body/Mind Therapies in Fox Chase, Philadelphia, PA, for twelve years.

For a complete Biography, Please visit
http://ReverendMikeWanner.com/Bio